I0104230

Stretching and Flexibility for Women

Womens Wellness Publishing, LLC
www.womenswellnesspublishing.com
www.facebook.com/wwpublishing

Mention of specific companies or products in this book does not suggest endorsement by the author or publisher. Internet addresses and telephone numbers for resources provided in this book were accurate at the time it went to press.

Cover design by Rebecca Rose

ISBN 978-1-939013-83-5

NOTE: The information in this book is meant to complement the advice and guidance of your physician, not replace it. It is very important that women who have medical problems be evaluated by a physician. If you are under the care of a physician, you should discuss any major changes in your regimen with him or her. Because this is a book and not a medical consultation, keep in mind that the information presented here may not apply in your particular case. In view of individual medical requirements, new research, and government regulations, it is the responsibility of the reader to validate health practices and treatments with a physician or health service.

Acknowledgements

I want to give a huge thanks to my amazing editors Kendra Chun and Sandra K. Friend for their incredibly helpful assistance with putting this book together. I also greatly appreciate my fantastic Creative Director, Rebecca Richards, as well as Letitia Truslow, my wonderful Director of Media Relations. I enjoyed working with all of them and found their help indispensable in creating this exceptional book for women. Most of all, I want to thank God and Jesus Christ for their love and blessings.

Table of Contents

1

How Stretching Can Change Your Life

Stretching exercises are a wonderful way to improve your flexibility and fitness. I recommend them to patients as part of my therapeutic programs to combat specific health issues and reduce pain and discomfort. In fact, most health conditions can benefit from doing a regular stretching program. Stretching enhances suppleness and elasticity of the joints, muscles and ligaments and improves circulation and oxygenation throughout the body. It can also help to balance mood and increase energy.

I have found that stretches enhance the youthfulness of the body and have significant anti-aging benefits. They help to prevent muscular stiffness, tightness and soreness that so many women suffer from. While stiffness, pain and discomfort are often seen in midlife and older women who are suffering from arthritis, fibromyalgia and the hormonal changes of menopause, even younger women are not immune to these symptoms.

I have worked with many younger women patients who were trying to deal with stiffness and soreness from too much deskwork and deadlines or even from engaging in rigorous physical activity. Food allergies and thyroid disease can also contribute to muscle tension, joint aching, pain and cramping in younger women.

One of my good friends, who I frequently go hiking with, is in her late twenties. She is very fit and exercises regularly, but she often complains to me about her shoulder and back pain from doing workouts that are too vigorous. Another one of my good friends complains of low back and hip pain, which concerns her since she is always chasing her small, active children around. Luckily, stretching routines can quite easily be worked into the busiest of schedules and help relax sore and aching muscles as well as provide a relaxing and energizing break from all of the "must dos" of the day.

One of the biggest culprits of pain and discomfort, at all ages, is emotional stress and tension. When we are feeling upset, no matter what the emotion, it is often reflected in our muscles, ligaments and tendons. The upset in our minds and feelings, whether fear, worry, anger, anxiety or depression, often translates into headaches, neck, shoulder, and arm pain, not to mention abdominal, hip and pelvic discomfort. Even calf and foot cramps can be exacerbated by stress and tension.

I have developed many different stretching routines, both for my patients and readers, over a number of years and decided that it would be wonderful to put them all together in one book that would be a great resource of women. These are routines that I also practice myself and I credit them for helping me to maintain a very flexible and supple body, despite all of the hours of desk and computer work that I do.

I make sure that I take stretching breaks several times a day and am thrilled that I have great range of motion of my joints and muscles. The stretches also remind me to take a deep breath, help me to relax and rejuvenate my energy.

I have included in this book stretching routines that I have developed for joint flexibility, total body fitness and flexibility, lower body flexibility, as well as a wonderful energizing sequence. These are stretches that were developed to increase your level of energy and vitality and enhance your sense of joy and calm.

I have also included very helpful exercise questionnaires which you may want to fill out before starting a stretching routine, as well as, helpful suggestions on how to motivate yourself and begin a stretching program.

You can choose the stretching programs that appeal to you the most and seem to provide the most benefits for your specific health and fitness needs. You can do my routines in combination with other exercise programs that you are already doing or you can do them by themselves.

These stretching routines can quite easily be worked into the busiest of schedules and provide a great break from the deskwork that so many of us do. I have included specific, detailed instructions that are easy to follow on how to do each stretch. I have also included pictures that illustrate how each stretch should be done. I hope that you enjoy my programs and find that they enhance your suppleness and flexibility!

2

Self-Evaluation and Motivation

In this chapter, I have included three questionnaires to pinpoint your current exercise habits; determine where you tend to localize muscle tension in your body; as well as identify symptoms that you may be suffering that reflect lack of physical fitness and stamina. You may find it helpful to take a few minutes to fill out these questionnaires.

Sometimes, we have the best intentions in the world to begin an exercise program but find it difficult to "get ourselves going", to motivate ourselves to take the first step. I have also included in this chapter helpful suggestions on how to motivate yourself to start a stretching program as well as how to begin your program. So let's start now!

Evaluating Your Fitness Level

If you are currently making the transition from a sedentary lifestyle to a regular exercise program, I recommend that you evaluate your level of fitness. If you have not already done so, I recommend that you fill out the following questionnaires on your current exercise habits, patterns of muscle tension, and symptoms of lack of physical fitness.

It is important to know if you have any undiagnosed medical problems that could affect your proper level of activity. These would include problems like thyroid disease, anemia, high blood pressure and hypo-glycemia, which can affect your exercise tolerance. I have had patients with thyroid imbalance, for example, who felt more anxious and short of breath when exercising, because their excessive levels of thyroid hormone were elevating their heart and pulse rates to unhealthy levels during times of increased activity.

If you find you have chronic muscle tension or feel out-of-breath after walking up a flight of stairs, you may actually have an underlying problem like anemia (low red blood cell count) or thyroid disease, which can often go undiagnosed if the symptoms are merely attributed to a sedentary lifestyle. In fact, I suggest that you share your responses to these questionnaires with your health-care provider because they may offer valuable clues to help discover a medical problem that hasn't yet been diagnosed.

Key to Exercise Habits. Exercise is a good outlet for stress and can improve oxygenation and reduce pain. If your total number of exercise periods per week is less than three, you will probably be more prone to multiple health issues, including obesity, PMS and menopause related symptoms, arthritis, high blood pressure, chronic fatigue and depression.

If you are exercising more than three times a week, keep doing your exercises; they are probably making your symptoms less severe. You may want to add the stretches included in this book to your present regime.

Exercise Habits

Check off the number of times you do any of the following:

Activity	Never	1x a Month	1 - 2x a Week	>2x a Week
Jogging				
Walking				
Bicycling				
Skiing				
Swimming				
Aerobic dancing				
Jumping rope				
Ice skating				
Roller skating				
Handball				
Racquetball				
Tennis				
Soccer				
Basketball				
Baseball				
Table tennis				
Golf				
Croquet				
Bowling				
Stretching				
Weight lifting				
Gardening				

Key to What Stress Does to Your Body. This evaluation should help you to become aware of where you store stress in your body. Everyone has her own favorite area: tensions automatically accumulate there, like nuts in a squirrel's cheek. This accumulation increases your general level of fatigue and lowers your energy. Storing tension in the spine can worsen cramps; storing it in the neck can cause headaches.

Try to remain aware of the areas where you store tension. When you feel tension building up in them, begin deep breathing. Often this will release the tension immediately.

What Stress Does to Your Body

Check the places where tension most commonly localizes in your body:

- o Shoulders
- o Neck and Throat
- o Grinding Teeth
- o Lower Back
- o Headache
- o Eyestrain
- o Arms
- o Stomach Muscles

Symptoms of Lack of Physical Fitness and Stamina

Check those symptoms that pertain to you:

	Yes	No
Fatigue, tiredness, lethargy		
Tiredness or exhaustion when walking less than a mile		
Shortness of breath when walking less than a mile		
Tiredness or exhaustion when walking up a flight of stairs		
Shortness of breath when walking up a flight of stairs		
Excessive weight or obesity		
Poor muscle tone		
Excessive muscle tension and/or cramping when engaging in physical activity		
Eyestrain		
Chronic neck pain and muscle tension		
Chronic shoulder and upper-middle-back tension		
Grinding of teeth (bruxism)		
Chronic low back pain		
Chronic abdominal tension		
Chronic arm tension		

Key to Lack of Physical Fitness and Stamina. If you find that symptoms listed in this evaluation pertain to you, you should start a stretching and flexibility program slowly and carefully. Your level of physical activity should be increased gradually until your body is more conditioned to the point where the stretches are not as difficult to do. You may want to notify your physician regarding these symptoms if they are causing you distress as some of these symptoms may indicate an underlying health problem that should be evaluated.

Motivating Yourself to Do a Stretching Program

If you encounter mental obstacles to beginning and sticking with a regular stretching program, there are many ways to overcome this resistance. It is helpful for you to pinpoint the exact cause of your resistance; this will make it easier to eliminate it.

- Make sure you do your stretching program at the time of day that feels most natural. For example, if you are a late riser, don't try to exercise early in the morning. Exercise when you are the least stressed and hurried by your schedule. If your largest amount of free time is in the late afternoon between work and dinner, put aside that time to engage in physical activity.

- Do your stretches in an attractive setting. Some women enjoy stretching in a quiet area of their home while other women like to do their stretches outside in their yard or a park, weather permitting.

- You may want to do your stretches with your partner, a friend or support person. This can be a great help in motivating and encouraging you to begin and stick with a stretching program.

- Use your mind to disconnect from your daily activities. Positive mental exercises can help you to relax before starting physical activity. Many women find that a few minutes of doing visualizations (seeing themselves performing and enjoying the stretching routine in their minds) or saying affirmations (positive statements about the benefits of exercise) prepares them for their stretching routine.

- Listen to music while you do stretches. Many women find that the exercise period goes by much more quickly and the process is more fun and enjoyable when they listen to music. Be sure to choose music that is mellow and relaxing as it will help improve your mood and relax you further.

- Be sure to choose stretches that appeal to you and that you enjoy. Don't do stretches that worsen your stress level or that you find boring.

Beginning a Stretching Program

Before you begin your stretching program read through the following guidelines. They will help you to perform your stretching program in an optimal manner. These guidelines are particularly good for women who are just beginning a stretching program after leading a sedentary life. They are also helpful for women who have previously been fit and active but stopped exercising because physical exertion, including stretching, seemed to worsen their fatigue or muscle tension. A stretching program, or any other exercise routine, that is too strenuous can leave a woman feeling more tense, uptight or tired than usual.

During the first week or two of your program, build up your exercise level gradually. Limit your initial stretching workouts to short sessions. For example, you might start out exercising every other day for only a few minutes. Then, increase the length of your sessions gradually in 5-minute increments until you are at the level that suits you the best.

How to Avoid Trauma or Injury

- Perform the stretches in a relaxed and unhurried manner. Be sure to set aside adequate time so you do not feel rushed. Anytime you feel discomfort or excessive muscle tension, stop doing the exercise. Then reevaluate your pace to see if it is too vigorous.

- Only do stretches that seem to be appropriate for your level of health or fitness. Do not do stretches that could promote injury to a part of your body that is already compromised. Choose stretches that, instead, seem to be appropriate for your level of health and fitness.

- If you have any questions about doing a particular set of stretches, I recommend that you check with your physician or health care provider to make sure that they approve before starting a program.

- Avoid doing stretches, or exercising, when you are ill or during times of extreme stress. At such times, the stress-reduction exercises or breathing exercises will be more useful.

- Move slowly and carefully when first starting to do a stretching program. This will help promote flexibility of the muscles and prevent injury. Follow the breathing instructions provided in the exercise. Most important, do not hold your breath. Allow your breath to flow in and out easily and effortlessly.

- Always rest for a few minutes after finishing a session.

- If you experience any pain or discomfort, you have probably over-reached your current ability and should immediately reduce the amount of the stretching until you can proceed without discomfort. Be careful, as muscular injuries can take quite a while to heal. If you do strain a muscle, I have found that immediately applying ice to the injured area for 10 minutes is quite helpful. Continue to use the ice pack two to three times a day for several days. If the pain persists, see your doctor.

3

General Fitness and Flexibility Exercises

The following exercises will promote mobility, flexibility, and relaxation. You can use them with great benefit to help loosen the joints in your lower body and decrease muscle stiffness and tension.

If you are in midlife or beyond, you may have more stiffness and lack of flexibility from the diminished production of female hormones that occurs when women enter menopause. These exercises can be extremely beneficial to help improve suppleness and elasticity of your muscles, ligaments and tendons.

Practiced on a regular basis, these exercises will also improve your vigor and energy level. You can use them to warm up tense and tight muscles before engaging in sports or athletic events.

I do many of these exercises myself and have found them to be very helpful during times of physical and emotional stress and tension. They have helped me tremendously to stay loose and flexible with my own self-care program.

How to Perform the General Fitness and Flexibility Exercises

- I recommend that you try all of these exercises during the first week or two of your program. However, if any of the exercises seem too difficult for your level of fitness, then it is best not to do those.

- Then put together your own routine based on the exercises that provide the most benefit. You may find that you want to use all of them on a regular basis, or perhaps only a few. The types of stretches included in my program can be very beneficial when used before any sports or athletic events.

- The stretches should be performed in a relaxed and unhurried manner. Be sure to set aside adequate time-30 minutes or more—so that you do not feel rushed. Your exercise area should be quiet, peaceful, and uncluttered.

- Wear loose, comfortable clothing. It's better to exercise without socks to give your feet complete freedom of movement and to prevent slipping.

- Wait at least two hours after eating to exercise. Evacuate your bowels or bladder before you begin the exercises.

- Choose a flat area and work on a mat or a blanket. This will make you more comfortable while you do the exercises.

- Pay close attention to the initial instructions when beginning an exercise. Look at the placement of the body as shown in the photographs. This is very important, for you are much more likely to have relief from your symptoms if you practice the exercise properly.

- Try to visualize the exercise in your mind, follow with proper placement of the body. This will help promote flexibility of the muscles and prevent injury. Follow the breathing instructions provided in the exercise. Most important, do not hold your breath. Allow your breath to flow in and out easily and effortlessly

- Move slowly through the exercise. This will help promote flexibility of the muscles and prevent injury. If you practice these stretches regularly in a slow, unhurried fashion, you will gradually loosen your muscles, ligaments, and joints. You may be surprised at how supple you can become over time.

- Always rest for a few minutes after doing the exercises. Try to practice these movements on a regular basis. A short session every day is best. If that is not possible, then try to practice them every other day.

Joint Motion and Flexibility

Exercise 1

Gentle range of motion exercises help to loosen tense muscles where they insert and originate near the joints. These are great stretches for any woman suffering from arthritis, fibromyalgia or stiffness and poor mobility. They are very useful for women who spend hours in front of the computer or doing deskwork where the range of motion of the muscles, ligaments and tendons is limited for long periods of time. This can lead to shortening and contracture of the muscle groups.

The following sequence produces a gentle stretching of the muscles around the joints, which will help to reduce tension and stress. These stretches are also thought to stimulate the acupuncture meridians. They are wonderful stretches for women who want to keep their joints and muscles mobile, elastic and supple. They are beneficial for every woman, no matter your age or stage of life.

Sit on the floor with your legs stretched out in front. Place your hands at your sides

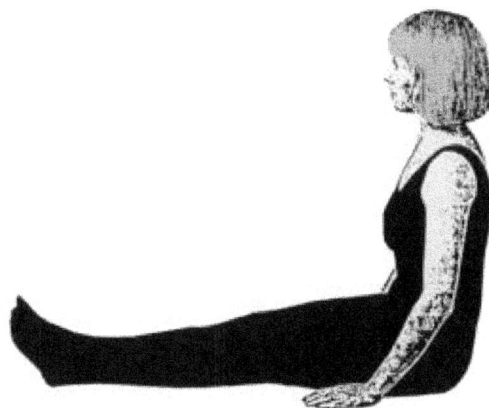

Toes: Slowly flex and extend the toes without moving your feet or ankles. Repeat 10 times.

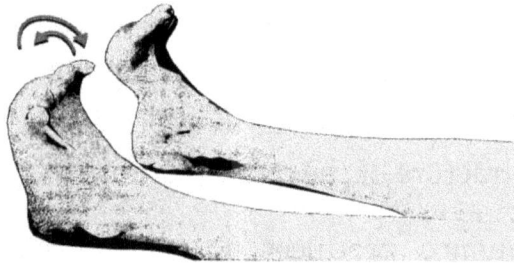

Ankles: Slowly flex and extend the ankle joints. Repeat 10 times. Separate your legs slightly, then rotate your ankles in each direction 10 times. Be sure to keep your heels on the floor.

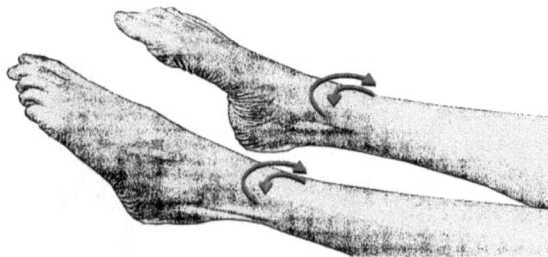

Knees: Still resting in the sitting position, bend the right leg at the knee, bringing the heel near the right buttock. Then lift the right leg off the floor, straightening the right knee. Repeat 10 times. Then do the same exercise with the left leg.

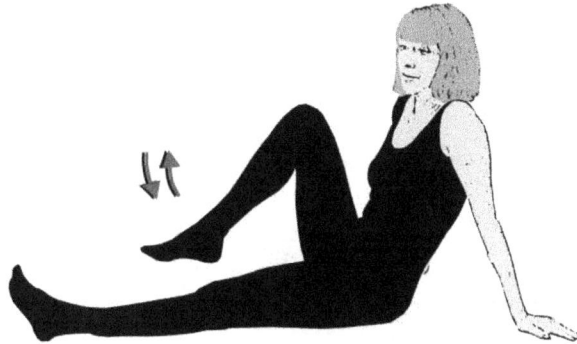

Hold the thigh near the chest with both hands. Rotate your lower leg in a circular motion about the knee 10 times clockwise and then 10 times counterclockwise. Repeat with the left leg.

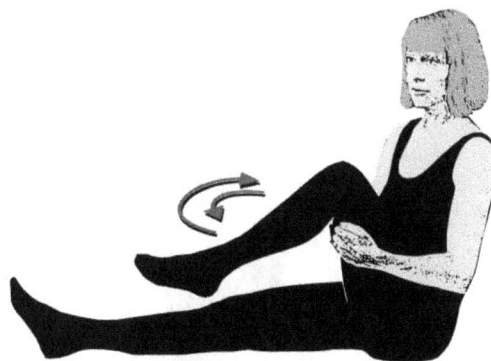

Hips: Bend the right leg so that you can place your right foot on the left thigh. Hold the right knee with the right hand and hold the right ankle with the left hand. Then gently move the right knee up and down with the right hand. Repeat with the left leg.

While you are sitting in the same position, rotate the right knee clockwise 10 times and then counterclockwise 10 times. This improves the flexibility of the hip joints. Repeat on the left side

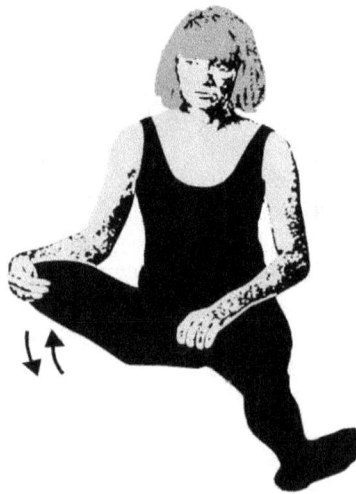

While sitting, bring the soles of the feet together, bringing the heels close to the body. Using your hands, gently push the knees to the floor and then let them come up again. Repeat 10 times.

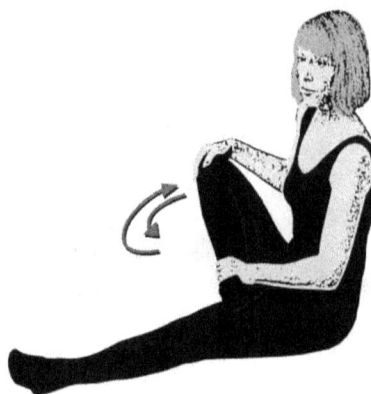

Spine: Remain sitting with your legs together straight out in front of you. Reach over and touch your legs or, without straining, your toes without bending your knees. Repeat 10 times.

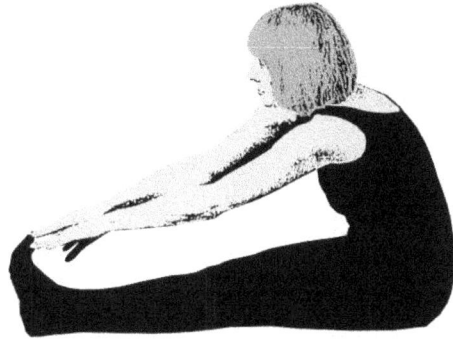

Fingers: Sit on the floor with your legs stretched out in front of you. Lift your arms up to shoulder height, keeping them straight. Open your hands wide. Flex the fingers, closing them over the thumbs to make a fist. Repeat 10 times

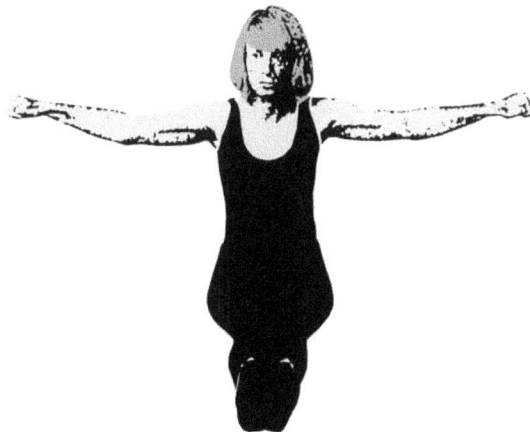

Wrists: Flex and extend your wrists. Repeat 10 times.

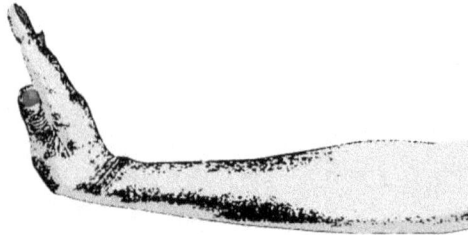

Sitting in the same position, rotate your wrists clockwise and counterclockwise. Repeat 10 times.

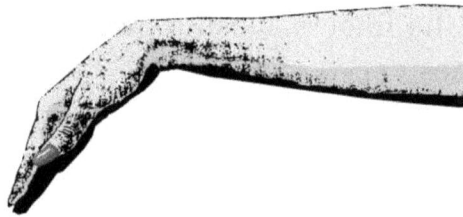

Sitting in the same position, hold your hands in extension and move each hand from side to side at the wrist. Repeat 10 times.

Elbows: Remaining in the same position, stretch out your arms at shoulder height with the palms facing upward.

Then bend your arms at the elbow so that your fingers touch the shoulders, and straighten out your arms again.

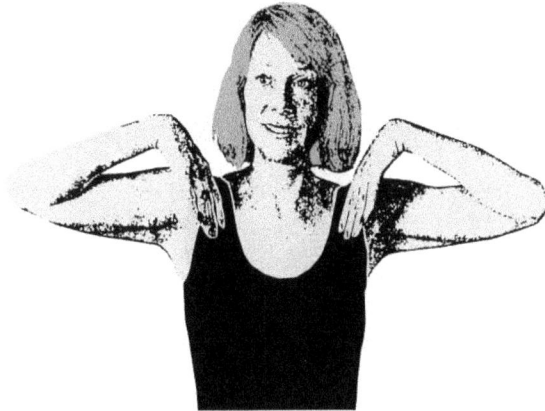

Repeat 10 times with arms extended sideways and ten times with arms facing forward.

Shoulders: From the same sitting position, with your arms bent and fingertips touching the shoulders, make a circular motion with your elbows. Repeat 10 times clockwise and 10 times counterclockwise.

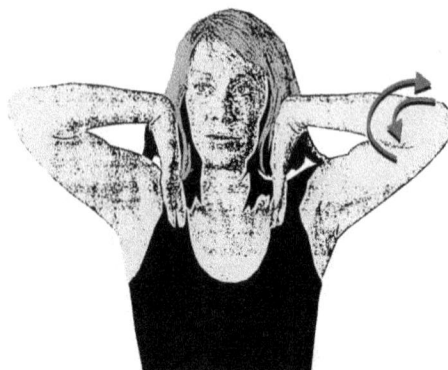

Spine: Remain sitting with your legs together straight out in front of you. Reach over and touch your legs or, without straining, your toes without bending your knees. Repeat 10 times.

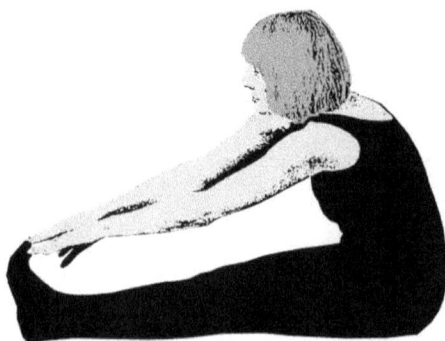

Waist: Stand up and slowly reach over and touch your lower legs or, without straining, your toes as you bend at the waist. Try to keep your knees straight.

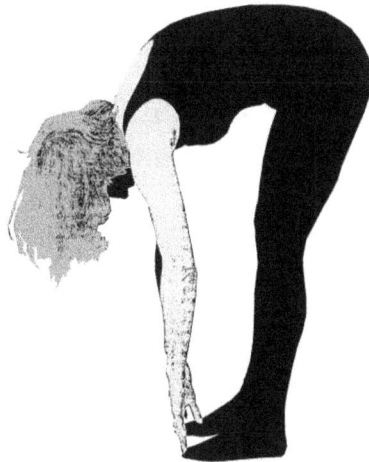

Repeat 10 times. If you have lower back problems do these two positions with caution

Total Body Flexibility Exercises

Exercise 1

This exercise improves circulation to the upper half of the body while energizing and stimulating it. It also loosens and stretches tense muscles in the upper body, especially the shoulders and back, and expands the lungs.

Stand easily. Arms should be at your sides; feet are hip distance apart. Bring your arms back slowly and gracefully until you can clasp them behind your back.

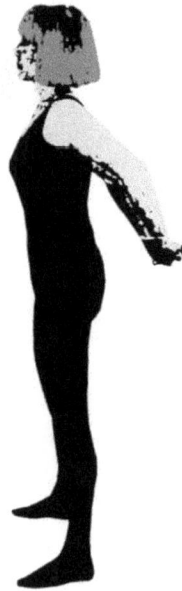

Exhale, then straighten your clasped hands and arms as far as you can without discomfort. Remember to stand upright; body should not bend forward. Breathe deeply into chest.

As you hold your breath, bend forward at the waist, bringing your clasped hands and arms up over your back. Relax your neck muscles and keep your knees straight.

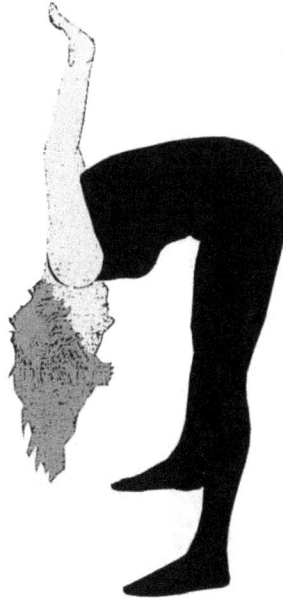

Hold for a few seconds. Exhale as you return to the upright position. Unclasp your hands and allow your arms to rest easily at your sides. Repeat entire sequence 3 times.

Exercise 2

This exercise relieves stiffness and tension in the neck, lubricates the vertebrae, and strengthens the muscles of the neck. You may want to repeat this exercise several times a day if your neck is particularly stiff. You may hear a gritty sound at first. This can accompany stiff and contracted muscles. Visualize your neck rolling slowly and smoothly on ball bearings as you do this exercise.

Sit in a chair with your arms and shoulders relaxed. First breathe in deeply, then exhale and allow your head to come all the way forward to your chest, keeping the spine straight. Hold for a few breaths.

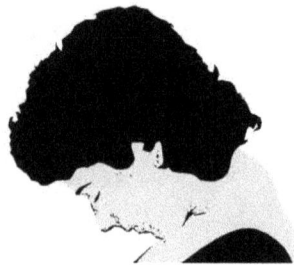

Exhale and bring your right ear to the right shoulder, keeping the right shoulder completely relaxed. Hold for a few breaths.

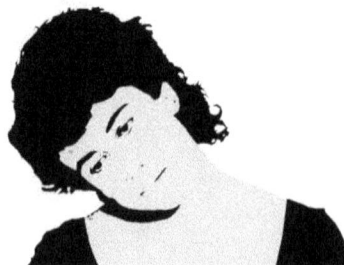

Exhale and allow your head to drop back, keeping the spine straight and the shoulders relaxed. Hold for a few breaths.

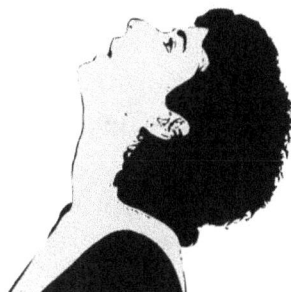

Bring your left ear to the left shoulder, keeping your left shoulder relaxed. Hold for a few breaths. Bring your head to the original position, keeping your chin forward. Slowly repeat the exercise moving in the opposite direction.

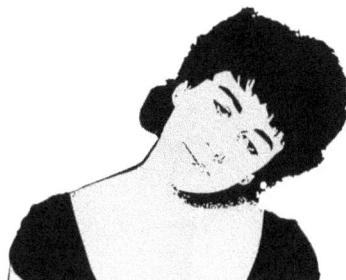

Exercise 3

This exercise relieves tension in the hips and shoulders, strengthens the legs and back, and aids in balance.

Stand easily with your arms at your sides. Raise your right arm slowly overhead. Shift your weight to your right leg.

Catch your left ankle with your left hand, bending leg at the knee. You will be balancing yourself on your right leg.

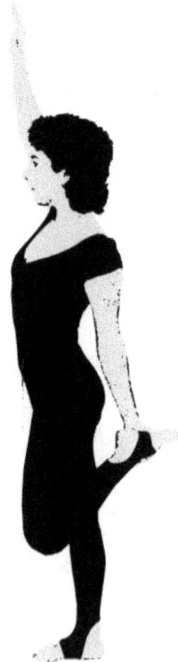

Gently stretch your back by bringing your right hand back a few inches and pulling your left leg up a few inches and moving it away from your body. This should be done slowly. The left arm remains straight to open the shoulder.

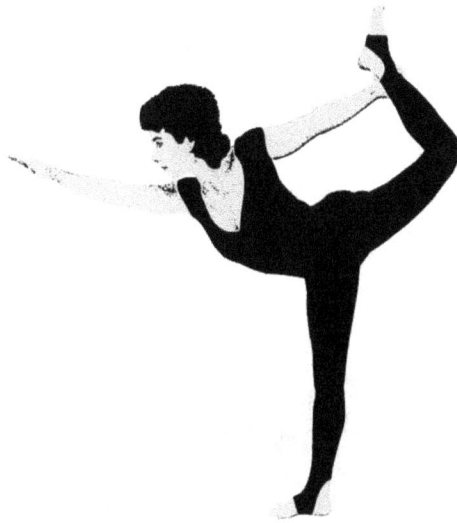

Slowly return to your original resting position. Repeat exercise on opposite foot.

Exercise 4

This exercise massages the entire neck and spine and flexes the vertebral column. It will invigorate and energize you, reducing fatigue.

Lie on your back. Bend and raise your knees to your chest, clasping them with your hands. Hands should be interlocked below knees.

Raise your head toward your knees and gently rock back and forth on your curved spine.

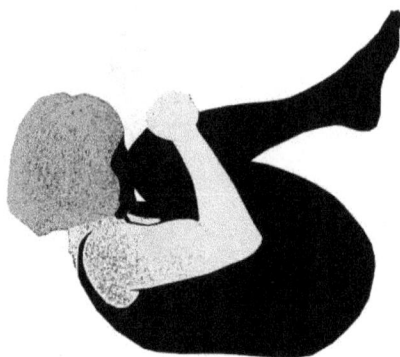

Note the roundness of your back and shoulders. Keep the chin tucked in as you roll back. Avoid rolling back too far on your neck. Rock back and forth 5 to 10 times.

Exercise 5

This exercise strengthens the back and abdominal muscles, improves blood circulation through the pelvis, and calms anxiety and nervousness.

Lie down and press the small of your back into the floor. This permits you to use your abdominal muscles without straining your lower back.

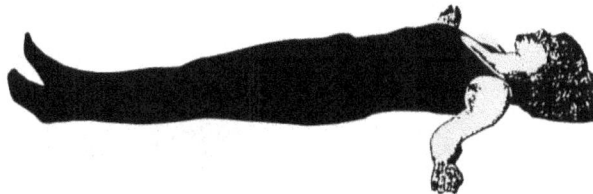

Keep your back flat on the floor and let the rest of your body remain relaxed.

Raise your right leg slowly while breathing in. Move your leg very slowly; imagine your leg being pulled up smoothly by a spring. Do not move your leg in a jerking manner. Hold for a few breaths.

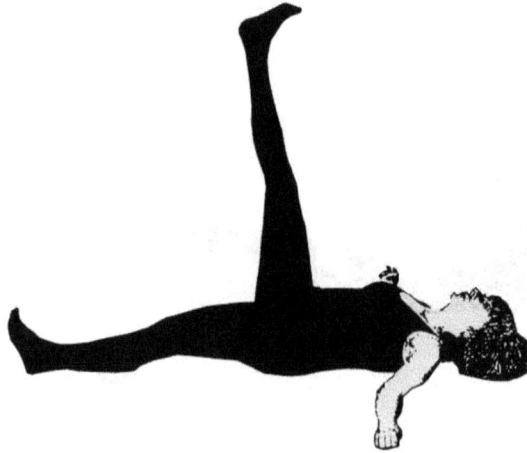

Lower your leg and breathe out. Repeat the same exercise on your left side. Then alternate legs, repeating the exercise 5 to 10 times.

Exercise 6

This exercise emphasizes freer pelvic movement with controlled breathing, energizes and rejuvenates the female reproductive tract, and tones the abdominal organs (pancreas, liver, and adrenals). It may also help relieve carbohydrate craving and dizziness.

Lie on your back with your knees bent and your feet on the floor close to your buttocks.

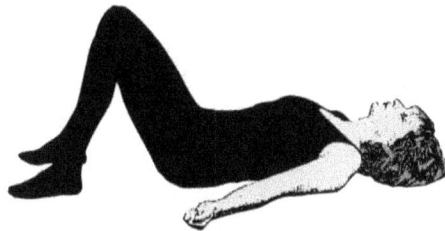

Exhale and press the lower back into the floor, raising the buttocks slightly.

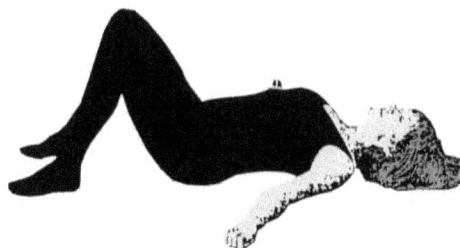

Arch the back slightly. Inhale and lift your lower back off the floor. This stretches the region from the sternum to the pelvis.

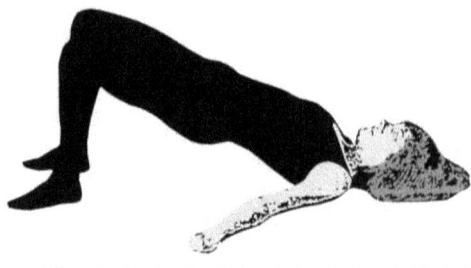

Repeat this exercise 10 times. Always lift your navel up on the in-breath. Always elongate your spine and press the lower back down on the out-breath.

Exercise 7

This exercise helps release overall body tension. It improves circulation and concentration. It strengthens the lower back and abdominal area.

Lie on your stomach with your feet together and your arms lying flat at your sides.

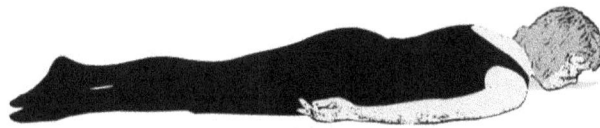

Stretch your arms out straight in front of you on the floor.

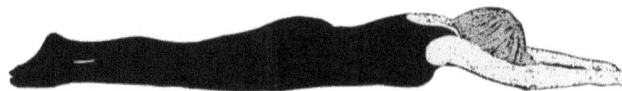

As you inhale, arch your back and lift your arms, head, chest and legs off the floor.

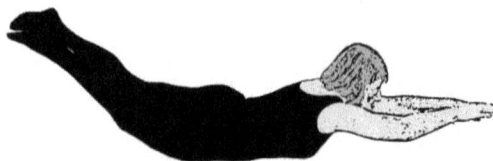

Hold the pose as long as you can, up to 30 seconds, breathing deeply and slowly.

Return to the original resting position with your head turned to the side, and completely relax for 1 to 3 minutes.

Exercise 8

This exercise is one of the most powerful stretches for increasing total body energy and vitality and releasing muscle tension. It strengthens the nervous system, balances the mood, may reduce sugar craving, and helps reduce anxiety and nervous tension. It improves concentration and mental clarity. It also stimulates the thyroid, thymus, liver, kidneys, and female reproductive tract, and improves digestive function.

Lie face down on the floor, arms at your sides. Slowly bend your legs at the knees and bring your feet up toward your buttocks.

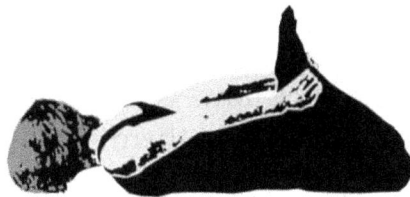

Reach back with your arms and carefully take hold of first one foot and then the other. Flex your feet to make grasping them easier.

Inhale and raise your trunk from the floor as far as possible. Lift your head and elevate your knees off the floor.

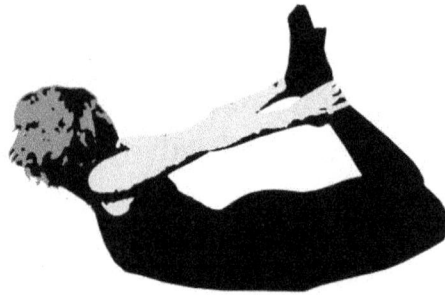

Squeeze the buttocks. Imagine your body looking like a gently curved bow. Hold for 10 to 15 seconds.

Slowly release the posture. Allow your chin to touch the floor and finally release your feet and return them slowly to the floor. Return to your original position. Repeat 5 times.

Lower Body Flexibility Exercises

Exercise 1: Muscle Tension Relaxation

This exercise is excellent for releasing muscle tension and improving circulation in the lower body. It stretches the muscles in the pelvis and lower back. Many women who do this exercise also notice an increase in their energy level. You may have a feeling of vitality upon completing this sequence. The pelvic movements are particularly helpful in bringing optimal blood flow, oxygen, and nutrients to this region, which may help relieve cramps, low back pain, and abdominal tension. Do the steps slowly and never do them so hard as to cause a strain or injury.

Stand with your legs spread apart about two feet. Point your feet out at a comfortable angle. Bend your knees slowly and lower your buttocks. Eventually, they should be able to go as low as your knees. Move up and down 10 times. Then, rock your pelvis back and forth in a swinging motion.

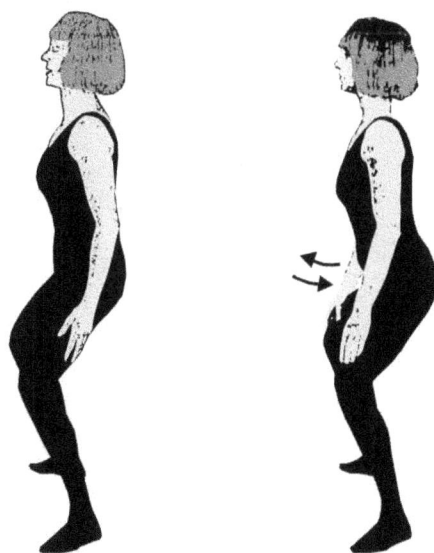

Move your hips and pelvis from side to side. Let your torso and arms sway in the opposite direction, as if dancing.

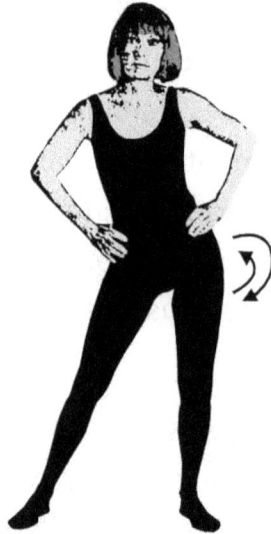

Then, move your hips around in a full circle. Do this several times in one direction and then the other.

Exercise 2: Lower Back Arch

This exercise helps loosen up the lower back muscles and promotes flexibility of the spine. It can also combat tiredness in women who experience deceased energy during the onset of menstruation.

Stand with your legs spread apart 1 foot. Point your feet straight ahead.

Place your hands around your waist with your thumbs pressing into your lower back

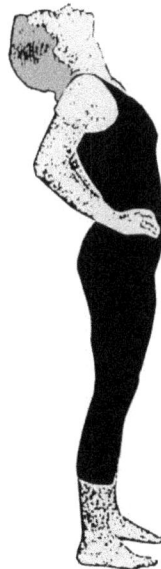

As you inhale, curve your back into an arch with your head held back. Place your hands around your waist with your thumbs pressing into your lower back.

As you exhale, let the weight of your body bend you forward so that your head almost touches your knees.

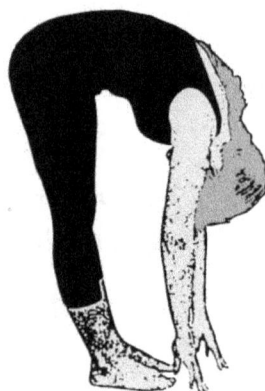

Hold for a few seconds. Do this exercise slowly and repeat several times.

Exercise 3: Abdominal Muscle Release

This exercise helps to release lower and upper abdominal tension. Many women with menstrual cramps often have digestive symptoms such as nausea and bowel changes. This twist helps to reduce the tension in the abdominal muscles that can worsen these symptoms.

Sit on the floor with your legs out in front. Place your hands on your shoulders with your fingers in front and thumbs in back.

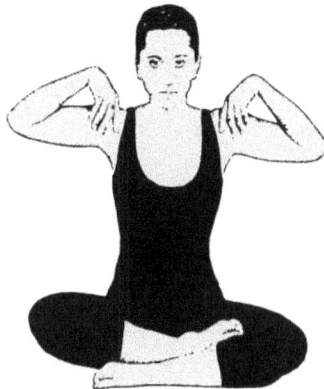

Be sure to keep your spine straight and inhale deeply.

As you inhale, twist your head, chest, and abdomen to the left. As you exhale, twist your body to the right.

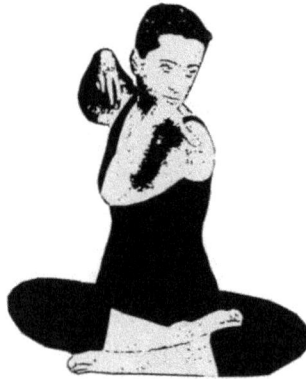

Do this exercise 4 times. Then reverse directions and repeat the sequence.

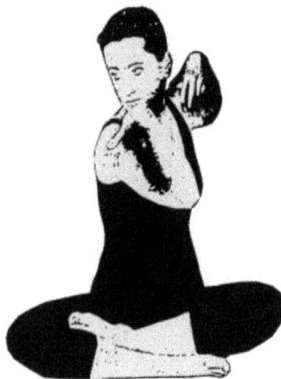

Exercise 4: Low Back Release

This exercise promotes relaxation, specifically in the lower back, hips, and abdominal muscles. By tensing and then releasing the abdominal and hip muscles, along with controlled heavy breathing, the entire mid- and lower body become looser and more supple. You may also notice a decrease in anxiety and emotional tension by the end of this exercise.

Lie on your back with your legs together. Raise your feet 6 to 8 inches off the ground; then raise your head and shoulders 6 inches, also.

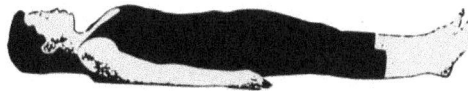

Point to your toes with your fingertips, keeping your arms straight and your eyes fixed on your toes. Then, breathe through your nose deeply to a count of 20.

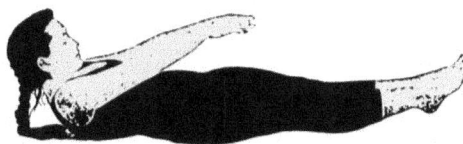

Lower your legs and head and relax. Rest for a count of 30. Repeat this exercise several times.

Exercise 5: Low Back Twist

This exercise allows you to twist over to the side, which is actually a natural position for your body to assume when you are feeling pelvic discomfort. This gentle stretch helps to lengthen the muscles in the low back as well as along the entire spine. It also helps to align the lumbar spine. Many women find that this exercise helps relieve pelvic tension and discomfort.

Lie on your back with your knees bent, feet placed flat on the floor.

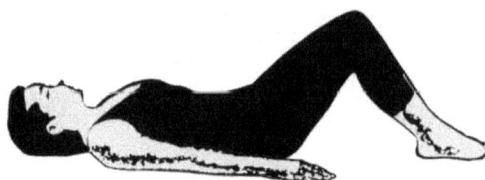

As you exhale, slowly let your knees and hips fall to the left as you turn your head to the right. Inhale and bring your knees back together to the center.

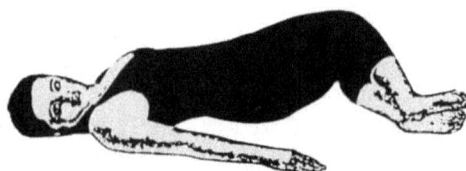

Then exhale again and reverse direction, letting your knees and hips fall to the right as you turn your head to the left.

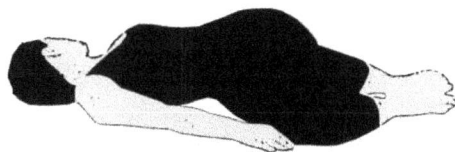

Repeat this exercise slowly several times, alternating sides.

Energizing Stretches

Exercise 1: Deep Breathing

Deep, slow abdominal breathing is essential for women to boost energy and vitality. It expands your lungs and allows you to bring adequate oxygen, the fuel for metabolic activity, to all the tissues of your body. Rapid, shallow breathing decreases your oxygen supply and keeps you tired and devitalized. Deep breathing helps to relax the entire body and strengthens the muscles in the chest and abdomen. It helps to stabilize mood and reduce both depression and anxiety, so it is very important for emotional wellbeing.

Lie flat on your back with your knees pulled up. Keep your feet slightly apart. Try to breathe in and out through your nose.

Inhale deeply. As you breathe in, allow your stomach to relax so that the air flows into your abdomen. Your stomach should balloon out as you breathe in. Visualize your lungs filling up with air so that your chest swells out.

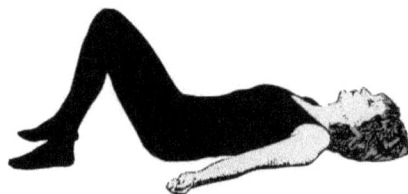

Imagine that the air you breathe is filling your body with energy

Exhale deeply. As you breathe out, let your stomach and chest collapse. Imagine the air being pushed out, first from your abdomen and then from your lungs.

Exercise 2: Total Body Muscle Relaxation

Women who are tired and devitalized tend to have poor muscle tone. They frequently have muscle groups that are tense and tight because of inadequate oxygenation and blood flow. Lactic acid tends to accumulate in these muscles, and muscle tension can become a chronic problem. Regular physical activity effectively breaks up this pattern of chronically tight muscles. Unfortunately, women who are tired and fatigued tend to become less active as their tiredness worsens.

Strenuous exercise is often too difficult for a woman who is combating fatigue, it is still very important to keep the muscles loose and flexible. Supple muscles definitely increase your level of energy and vitality. Flexible muscles also have a beneficial effect on mood and induce a sense of peace and calm. The following exercise helps you to get in touch with the parts of your body that feel tense and contracted. It will also aid in releasing muscle tension and restoring elasticity and flexibility.

Lie in a comfortable position. Allow your arms to rest limply, palms down, on the surface next to you.

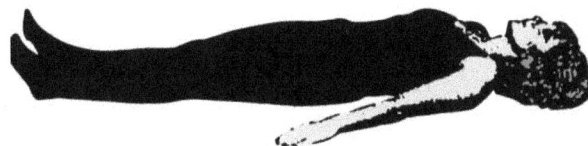

Breathe slowly and deeply as you do this exercise.

Raise your right hand off the floor and hold it there for 15 seconds. Notice any tension in your forearm or upper arm.

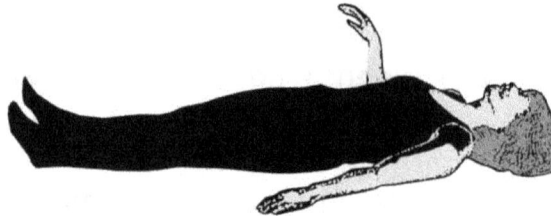

Let your hand slowly relax and rest on the floor. The hand and arm muscles should relax. As you lie there, notice any other parts of your body where you are carrying tension.

Clench your hands into fists and hold them tightly for 15 seconds. As you do this, relax the rest of your body. Then let your hands relax.

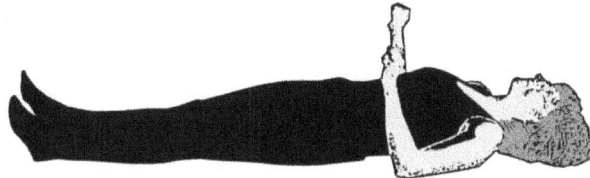

Now, tense and relax the following parts of your body in this order: face, shoulders, back, stomach, pelvis, legs, feet, and toes. Hold each part tensed for 15 seconds and then relax your body for 30 seconds before going on to the next part.

Visualize the tense part contracting, becoming tighter and tighter. On relaxing, see the energy flowing into the entire body like a gentle wave, making all the muscles soft and pliable.

Finish the exercise by shaking your hands. Imagine the remaining tension flowing out of your fingertips.

4

Energizing Sequence

This exercise sequence is excellent for increasing your energy, releasing muscle tension and improving circulation. Many women feel increased vitality and vigor upon completing this set. The exercises stimulate movement and energy flow through all muscles of the body, starting from the legs and moving up to the top of the head. In traditional Chinese healing models, these exercises are thought to stimulate the seven chakras or vital energy centers of the body.

Do the steps in this sequence slowly, to avoid stressing the body. As your strength and flexibility improve, you may want to do the steps a little more vigorously.

Legs and Hips

Sit on the floor with your legs stretched straight in front of you. Place your hands on the floor behind you. Lift your buttocks very slightly off the floor and balance gently on the base of your spine. Repeat 5 times.

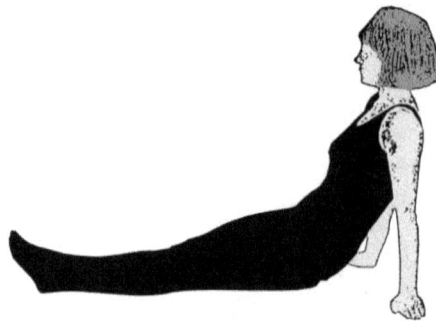

Legs and Pelvis

Stand with your legs spread apart about two feet. Point your feet out at a comfortable angle.

Bend your knees slowly and lower your buttocks. Eventually, they should be able to go as low as your knees.

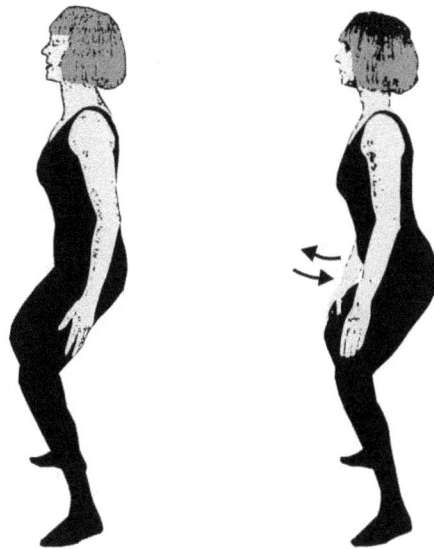

Move up and down 10 times. Then, rock your pelvis back and forth in a swinging motion.

Move your hips and pelvis from side to side. Let your torso and arms sway in the opposite direction, as if dancing.

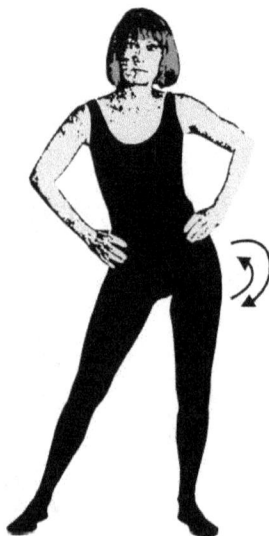

Then, move your hips around in a full circle. Do this several times in one direction and then the other.

Pelvis and Lower Abdomen

Lie on your stomach, placing your fists under your hips. Rest your forehead on the floor.

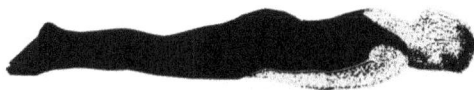

As you inhale, raise your right leg with an upward thrust, keeping your hips on your fists. Hold for 5 to 20 seconds if possible.

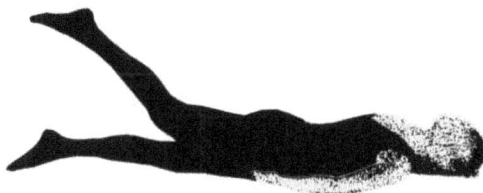

Lower the leg and slowly bring it back to the original position. Repeat several times. Then do the exercise on the left side.

Abdomen and Chest

Sit on your heels with your hands placed on your knees. As you inhale, arch your back and stretch to expand your chest up and out.

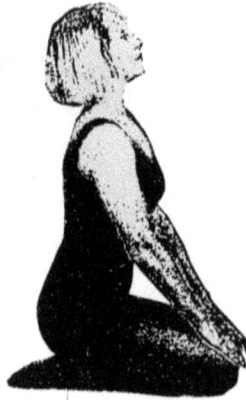

As you exhale, slump down to curve your back Repeat several times

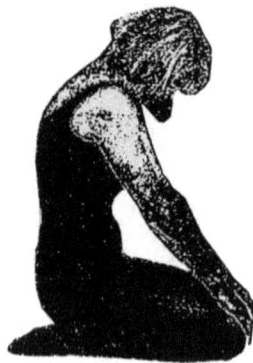

Abdomen and Shoulders

Sit on the floor with your legs out in front. Place your hands on your shoulders with your fingers in front and thumbs in back. Be sure to keep your spine straight and inhale deeply.

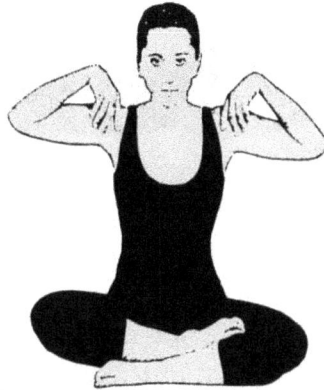

Turn your elbows, head, and neck to the left and then to the right.

Repeat 10 times. Be sure to let your entire torso move with your shoulders and arms.

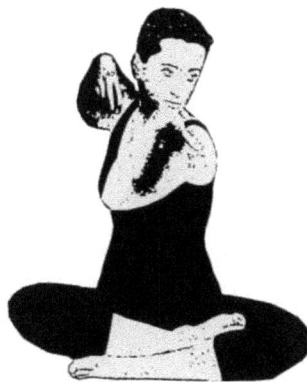

Back and Chest

Lean backward over a hassock or a big soft pillow, so that your chest opens and expands as your shoulders go backward.

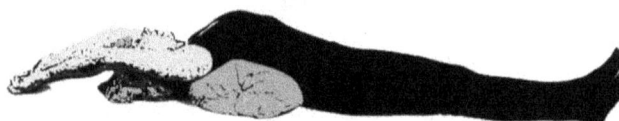

Let the muscles of your chest relax. Keep your feet firmly on the floor.

Neck

Sit on your knees with your hands on your thighs. Take a deep breath and stretch your body upward.

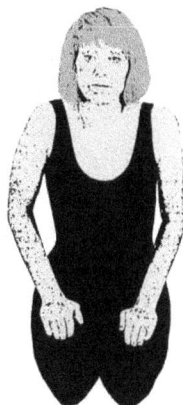

As you exhale, widen your eyes, stick out your tongue and push your body forward. Hold this position to the count of 10. Repeat this exercise 5 times.

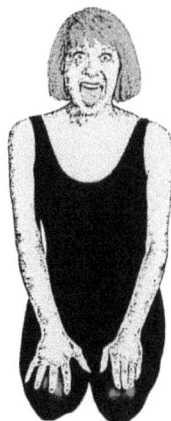

Neck

Lie flat on your back on the floor in a relaxed manner. As you inhale, slowly turn your head to the left. Then, exhale as you return your head to the center position.

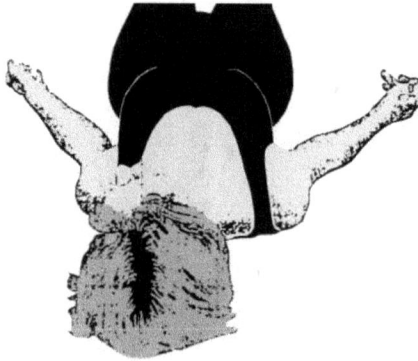

As you inhale again, turn your head to the right. Continue this exercise for 1 minute.

Eyes

With your head facing straight and your facial muscles relaxed, roll your eye muscles in the following directions: up and down, and side to side.

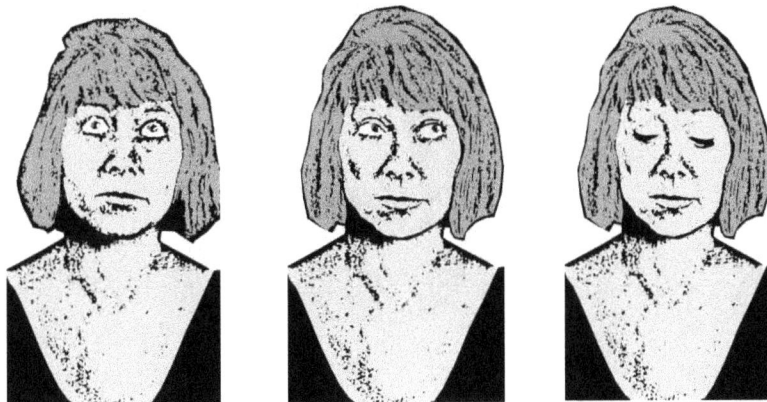

Move your eye muscles up to the left and down to the right. Reverse, moving your eyes up to the right and down to the left.

Head

Lie on your back. Your arms should be at your sides, palms up. Close your eyes and relax your whole body. Inhale and exhale slowly, breathing from the diaphragm.

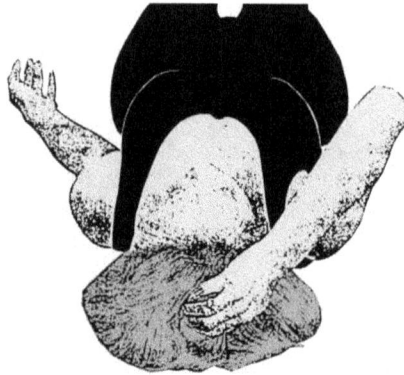

Rub the crown of your head in a clockwise motion with your right hand for 30 seconds.

About Susan M. Lark, M.D.

Dr. Susan Lark is one of the foremost authorities in the fields of women's health care and alternative medicine. Dr. Lark has successfully treated many thousands of women emphasizing holistic health and complementary medicine in her clinical practice. Her mission is to provide women with unique, safe and effective alternative therapies to greatly enhance their health and well-being.

A graduate of Northwestern University Feinberg School of Medicine, she has served on the clinical faculty of Stanford University Medical School, and taught in their Division of Family and Community Medicine.

Dr. Lark is a distinguished clinician, author, lecturer and innovative product developer. Through her extensive clinical experience, she has been an innovator in the use of self-care treatments such as diet, nutrition, exercise and stress management techniques in the field of women's health, and has lectured extensively throughout the United States on topics in preventive medicine. She is the author of many best-selling books on women's health. Her signature line of nutritional supplements and skin care products are available through healthydirections.com

One of the most widely referenced physicians on the Internet, Dr. Lark has appeared on numerous radio and television shows, and has been featured in magazines and newspapers including: Real Simple, Reader's Digest, McCall's, Better Homes & Gardens, New Woman, Mademoiselle, Harper's Bazaar, Redbook, Family Circle, Seventeen, Shape, Great Life, The New York Times, The Chicago Tribune, and The San Francisco Chronicle.

She has also served as a consultant to major corporations, including the Kellogg Company and Weider Nutrition International, and was spokesperson for The Gillette Company Women's Cancer Connection.

Dr. Lark can be contacted at (650) 561-9978 to make an appointment for a consultation.

We would enjoy hearing from you! Please share your success stories, requests for new topics and comments with us. Our team at Womens Wellness Publishing may be contacted at yourstory@wwpublishing.com. We invite you to visit our website for Dr. Lark's newest books at womenswellnesspublishing.com.

Dr. Susan's Solutions
Health Library For Women

The following books are available from Amazon.com, Amazon Kindle, iTunes, Womens Wellness Publishing and other major booksellers. Dr. Susan is frequently adding new books to her health library.

Women's Health Issues

Dr. Susan's Solutions: Heal Endometriosis

Dr. Susan's Solutions: Healthy Heart and Blood Pressure

Dr. Susan's Solutions: Healthy Menopause

Dr. Susan's Solutions: The Anemia Cure

Dr. Susan's Solutions: The Bladder Infection Cure

Dr. Susan's Solutions: The Candida-Yeast Infection Cure

Dr. Susan's Solutions: The Chronic Fatigue Cure

Dr. Susan's Solutions: The Cold and Flu Cure

Dr. Susan's Solutions: The Fibroid Tumor Cure

Dr. Susan's Solutions: The Irregular Menstruation Cure

Dr. Susan's Solutions: The Menstrual Cramp Cure

Dr. Susan's Solutions: The PMS Cure

Emotional and Spiritual Balance

Breathing Meditations for Healing, Peace and Joy

Dr. Susan's Solutions: The Anxiety and Stress Cure

Women's Hormones

DHEA: The Fountain of Youth Hormone

Healthy, Natural Estrogens for Menopause

Pregnenolone: Your #1 Sex Hormone

Progesterone: The Superstar of Hormone Balance

Testosterone: The Hormone for Strong Bones, Sex Drive and Healthy Menopause

Diet and Nutrition

Dr. Susan Lark's Healing Herbs for Women

Dr. Susan Lark's Complete Guide to Detoxification

Enzymes: The Missing Link to Health

Healthy Diet and Nutrition for Women: The Complete Guide

Renew Yourself Through Juice Fasting and Detoxification Diets

Energy Therapies and Anti-Aging

Acupressure for Women: Relieve Symptoms of Dozens of Health Issues Through Pressure Points

Exercise and Flexibility

Stretching and Flexibility for Women

Stretching Programs for Women's Health Issues

About Womens Wellness Publishing

"Bringing Radiant Health and Wellness to Women"

Womens Wellness Publishing was founded to make a positive difference in the lives of women and their families. We are the premier publisher of print and eBooks focused on women's health and wellness. We are committed to publishing the finest quality and most comprehensive line of books that covers every area that a woman needs to create vibrant health and a joyful, fulfilling life.

Our books are written and created by the top health and wellness experts who share with you, our readers, their wisdom and extensive experience successfully treating many thousands of patients.

We encourage you to browse through our online bookstore; new books are frequently being added at womenswellnesspublishing.com. Also visit our Lifestyle Center and Customer Bonus Center for more exciting and helpful health and wellness information and resources.

Follow us on Facebook for the latest health tips, recipes, and all natural solutions to many women's health issues (facebook.com/wwpublishing).

About Our Associate Program

We invite you to become part of the Womens Wellness Publishing Community through our Associate Program. You will have the opportunity to earn generous commissions on sales that you create through your blog, social network, support groups, community groups, school & alumni groups, friends, family or other networks.

To join our program, go to our website and click "Become an Associate" (womenswellnesspublishing.com). We support your sales and marketing efforts by offering you and your customers:

- Free support materials with updates on all of our new book releases, promotions, and bonuses for you and your customers
- Free audio downloads, booklets, and guides
- Special discounts and sales promotions